Values in Conflict
Resolving Ethical Issu[es]

Second Edition

American Hospital Association

AHA

ISBN 0-87258-668-5

Copyright© 1994 by the American Hospital Association

10M-04/94

Contents

Preface and Acknowledgments

Values in Conflict: Resolving Ethical Issues in Health Care was developed by the AHA Technical Panel on Biomedical Ethics and had as its base *Values in Conflict: Resolving Ethical Issues in Hospital Care*, which was written in 1985 by the AHA Special Committee on Biomedical Ethics, the technical panel's predecessor.

Although this version is the second edition, in many ways it is new. In the past decade, many hospitals and health care systems have demonstrated a strong commitment to grappling with and helping their communities to address the complex ethical dilemmas that arise in providing health care services. During the same period, the challenges have become more sophisticated, and additional issues have emerged. The technical panel hopes that this new version will further stimulate those who have already made biomedical ethics a priority and provide the impetus for others to develop policies, educational programs, and guidance mechanisms to assist in understanding and resolving value conflicts.

I am personally grateful to have had the privilege of chairing the special committee and the technical panel, both of which included an outstanding array of ethicists, clinicians, administrators, trustees, and health care professionals. Special thanks to Joanne Lynn, M.D., and Christine Mitchell, R.N., who have served with me on both bodies. I also want to recognize the thoughtful work and contributions of the other technical panel members: Jean Adnopoz, Nancy K. Green, Robert L. Harman, Bruce Jennings, Ruth Macklin, Ph.D., Robyn Shapiro, J. D., and Kenneth Shull. Special gratitude to the AHA staff members who have worked with the technical panel: Gail Lovinger and Kathy Poole, the exceptionally able staff to the technical panel; and Alexandra Gekas, Margaret Hardy, J.D., and Donald Phillips.

Finally, I wish to thank the AHA Board of Trustees and executive management for their support of the technical panel's work and for this second edition of *Values in Conflict*. It is the technical panel's hope that this publication will contribute to the Association's leadership in helping health care institutions and organizations address ethical issues with compassion, caring, and understanding.

Paul B. Hofmann
Chairman, Technical Panel on Biomedical Ethics
December 1993

Introduction

The first edition of *Values in Conflict: Resolving Ethical Issues in Hospital Care* was published almost ten years ago in response to the increasing complexity and number of ethical dilemmas in health care. The intervening period has witnessed an even greater acceleration of bioethical issues facing not only the medical and research community and health care providers and patients but also society as a whole. Progress has been made on many issues, but countless new dilemmas have arisen to take their place. The dilemmas, concerns, and questions have become almost daily topics in the media. They range from resource allocation and rationing to cloning, assisted suicide, right to live, and right to die. The same period has also witnessed the beginning of what promises to be fundamental change in the way health care is financed and delivered. Financing changes emphasize managing within fixed resources and ensuring cost-effective delivery of care. Delivery changes stem from a new emphasis on integration of services, continuity of care, and health status and community.

This second edition of *Values in Conflict: Resolving Ethical Issues in Health Care* attempts to consider both the changing bioethical environment and the changing health delivery environment.

By virtue of its mission, its historical roots in charitable and religious organizations, and its fiduciary commitment to each patient and community, the hospital has traditionally been perceived as having a particular, even if implicit, moral responsibility for health care. The emerging integrated health delivery organizations and networks, which include hospitals and other types of providers, inherit the legacy of these traditions.

As health care providers and as employers with a commitment to patient care, hospitals and networks must develop policies and mechanisms to address questions of human values. As centers of health care delivery in the community, hospitals and networks must respond responsibly to social problems and dilemmas that affect the demand and need for health care services. Because responsibilities include supervision and review of patient care, standards of quality must be met and the basic processes that characterize relationships and decisions between patients and health care professionals must be consistent with sound ethical principles.

These roles all reinforce the need for a coherent, systemwide approach to ethical issues that arise in health care. This report is intended as a guide for health care executives, trustees, physicians, nurses, ethics committee members, and other health care professionals. It identifies issues that should be considered in resolving values conflicts in delivery of patient care. Although it suggests approaches to resolving conflicts, for the most part it avoids prescribing specific structures or policies.

Making Patient Care Decisions

Decision making in medical care should not be viewed as a single event. Medical care is constructed of a series of decisions, each of which influences the decisions that follow. The patient is expected to make choices based on available information on treatment options; likely outcomes, risks, and side effects; and the relationship of potential decisions and their outcomes to the patient's values and preferences.

In retrospect, patient care decisions once seemed simpler. Physicians used their best judgment to decide the course of treatment from an extremely limited range of options. As medical capabilities advanced, as the spectrum of disease shifted toward chronic disease and conditions affecting the elderly, and as the values of society changed, this paternalistic approach began to give way to a decision-making model based on the patient's authority to direct his or her own health care. Patient self-determination was consistent with society's developing emphasis on consumerism and personal rights. However, the optimum decision-making process uses the expertise and experience of both the physician and the patient.

*Although the term *physician* is used, at times other health care professionals, particularly nurses, may be principals in the relationship.

The patient-physician relationship and the health care setting provide the context for most treatment decisions*. In the best of circumstances, both parties, as part of an ongoing relationship, have agreed explicitly or implicitly on how decisions should be made. Whether the physician or patient takes principal responsibility for decisions on medical care usually depends on the situation as well as the personality and preferences of both the physician and the patient. However, to the extent possible, the patient and the physician should reach these decisions collaboratively. Decisions should reflect evaluation of outcomes of alternative plans of care from the perspective of particular patient preferences.

In some cases, patients from different ethnic and cultural backgrounds may have different expectations concerning the role of the physician and family. These different perspectives should be respected and ordinarily be accommodated.

Collaborative Decision Making

A key ingredient of collaborative decision making is open and truthful communication between the physician and the patient. It relies on the physician's understanding and experience and the patient's self-awareness of personal values and goals. For optimal collaborative decision making, the physician should provide accurate information as completely as possible and should usually recommend a course of treatment that reflects sound medical judgment and an understanding of the patient. Treatment options should be considered within the context of likely outcomes and how those outcomes relate to the patient's values and preferences. A treatment that is welcomed by one patient may be the worst fear of another because of pain, disfigurement, or other outcomes or side effects. Physicians must be open to considering alternative courses of treatment in an effort to find an option most closely aligned with the patient's values. The patient should ask questions of the physician, seek information from other sources if needed, and provide the physician with information and insights into personal preferences and life-style that can help the physician in recommending procedures and therapy. As a result, both parties make the decision collaboratively.

Although the hospital does not have a major responsibility in this decision-making process, its policies should encourage collaborative decision making between the physician and the patient. The hospital should have policies and practices that support and safeguard all aspects of informed consent and collaborative decision making. These policies and practices must recognize that the unfamiliar and stressful hospital environment may impair the ability of patients to assert themselves in making decisions and seeking information. Emotional factors associated with being sick or injured may also hamper patient reasoning and decision-making capability. In addition, patients may lack the confidence and empowerment derived from normal relations with family and friends and participation in daily routines.

Informed Consent

Informed consent is often mistakenly viewed as merely obtaining a signature on a standard form. Informed consent is more accurately described as a communication process that results in the patient's voluntary decision based on an understanding of the proposed action and its purpose, benefits, risks, and alternatives. The signed informed consent form merely documents that some key elements of communication have taken place.

Consent is most often considered as agreement to a particular procedure or a set of routine procedures. A specific consent is usually required for surgery, other invasive procedures, or major diagnostic tests. However, a particular treatment decision or diagnostic procedure is only one element in an overall treatment plan and structure, which the patient must understand to give a fully informed consent. Whenever possible, the patient should have the opportunity to ask questions, request additional information, or consult with others as desired before making a treatment decision. Also, if the patient's health insurance limits the range of options, the patient is entitled to specific and timely information about the nature, costs, risks, and benefits of alternatives excluded from coverage.

Some hospitals ask patients to sign a general consent for routine procedures and practices upon admission. This general consent is not specific to the patient's condition or treatment plan or any procedures. It generally does not satisfy the ethical or legal obligations implicit in informed consent. Patients are entitled to information about the purpose, process, and effects of tests, medications, and examinations that are part of routine care and treatment. This communication is even more important in hospitals with house staffs and larger institutions where many persons may have responsibility for various aspects of the patient's care.

The Choice Not to Consent

State laws widely recognize and uphold the patient's right to choose not to have tests or therapeutic treatment, including life-sustaining treatment, and/or to elect to receive only palliative care. The institution must facilitate the exercise of this right within the context of the hospital's mission and state and federal law. When a patient has chosen not to pursue life-sustaining treatment, the self-interest of others—family, friends, and health care professionals—should not be permitted to compromise the patient's rights.

Like consent to treatment, refusal of a recommended treatment should be properly documented and subject to appropriate review. Decisions related to refusal of life-sustaining treatment should be consensual and result from information sharing and discussion among the attending physicians, other involved health care professionals, and the patient or the patient's surrogate/family.

Resources to Aid Decision Making

When possible, hospitals should assist patients who wish additional information or support in decision making. Hospital libraries or patient education departments may wish to have reading materials for patients or to have cooperative arrangements with other libraries to obtain information for patients. In addition, a number of individuals, including chaplains, social workers, patient representatives, and nurses, can provide information, counsel, and support to the patient in the decision-making process. If the patient agrees, information may also be shared with family members and others who are involved in the process.

Hospital Responsibilities in Informed Consent

Hospitals have three major responsibilities related to patient consent:

- Hospitals are responsible for ensuring that proper informed consent has been obtained for diagnostic and therapeutic procedures performed in the hospital. When multiple caregivers are directly involved in the patient's care, hospitals should develop procedures to ensure that communication with the patient on these issues is consistent and coordinated.
- Hospitals should support and, if necessary, develop education programs for the medical staff on effective ways to achieve ethically and legally acceptable informed consent. They may wish to encourage their medical staffs to develop guidelines to help physicians in the communication process. Such guidance should emphasize sensitivity to cultural differences and the educational background, knowledge, beliefs, language, and emotional condition of the patient. In addition, it should stress the importance of objective and unbiased presentation of information, including the physician's recommendation.
- Hospitals are responsible for informing patients of their rights to consent to or reject proposed procedures and treatments and to formulate advance directives. The Patient Self-Determination Act (see p. 14) requires that

hospitals distribute to patients on admission information on these issues prepared or approved by the state government. However, the hospital also should call these rights to the patient's attention in other materials, such as patient handbooks and hospital statements of patient rights and responsibilities.

Patient Decision-Making Capacity

Decision-making capacity requires the abilities to make and communicate a decision that reflects an understanding and appreciation of the nature and consequences of the proposed and alternative actions and to evaluate them in relation to personal preferences and priorities. Usually, there is little question as to the capacity or incapacity of a patient to make a valid decision. In other cases, however, physical and/or mental condition, effects of treatment, legal status, or psychological characteristics may limit the ability of patients to participate effectively. Decision-making capacity focuses only on the ability of an individual to function in decision-making situations and is not synonymous with the legal term *competence*.*

*The Hastings Center. *Guidelines on the Termination of Life-Sustaining Treatment and the Care of the Dying*. Bloomington: Indiana University Press, 1988.

Assessment of Capacity

In the absence of indicators to the contrary, hospitals and health care professionals should assume that any adult patient has adequate decision-making capacity. The determination of capacity should generally be based on the patient's ability to function in the context of the decisions to be made rather than an automatic determination based on other patient characteristics—for example, elderly or mildly demented. A patient's capacity to make a decision should not be judged solely by the content of that decision. Rejecting a physician's recommendation or selecting a high-risk alternative may well indicate that the patient's values differ from those of the physician or the general public.

The capacity to make *some* decisions should be distinguished from the capacity to make *all* decisions that may arise in the course of treatment. Even patients with limited capacity should be encouraged to make some decisions. Decision making in the health care institution extends beyond dramatic issues to decisions on routine X-rays and tests, need for pain medication, menu selection, and preferences in clothes. Enabling the patient to make as many of these decisions as possible shows respect for the patient and the patient's autonomy. Furthermore, participation in this type of decision making may well empower the patient and enhance the patient's capacity to make weightier choices. Physicians, nurses, other members of the health care team, and concerned family members should be encouraged to identify what types of decisions an individual with limited capacity can make. Hospitals, through ethics committees, medical staff committees, publications, or in-service education programs, can enhance this process by emphasizing the importance of involving patients in decision making.

In addition, an individual's capacity to make decisions on care and treatment may fluctuate during the course of an illness. Physicians and other caregivers should use periods of better decision-making capacity to discuss alternatives, advantages, and risks of proposed treatment, and to encourage the patient to indicate treatment preferences in advance.

Although the attending physician is principally responsible for assessing decision-making capacity, other members of the health care team and the patient's family and friends often can provide useful observations on the patient's decision-making capacity. The patient's nurse and other caregiving staff can observe the patient's behavior. Family and friends can recognize if the patient is behaving abnormally, or expressing preferences discordant with long-standing values. Health care professionals, family, and friends should be encouraged to talk with the attending physician about observable changes that may affect a patient's capacity for decision making.

In rare cases of strong disagreement about a patient's decision-making capacity, consultation with appropriate specialists, such as mental health professionals, may be helpful or necessary. Such consultation may also be necessary to obtain a legal determination of incompetence. It should be remembered, however, that assessments of a patient's capacity to make a decision apply to the immediate issue; they do not necessarily provide a long-term statement on the ability of the patient. Usually these assessments are informal, ongoing judgments aimed at determining whether the patient can make decisions that reflect his or her preferences and priorities.

As the patient's condition changes, assessments of capacity should be reviewed. If patients can understand information, they usually should be notified of concerns about their capacity and should be offered an opportunity for reassessment or access to institutional review mechanisms. Legal adjudication is also a possible recourse.

Sometimes, various barriers can hamper the patient's ability to understand the nature and effects of treatment options. Difficulty with the English language or hearing or visual impairments must not compromise the patient's decision-making role. The Americans with Disabilities Act requires hospitals to have an effective means of communicating with patients who are visually or hearing impaired. The hospital should also see to it that, whenever possible, staff or volunteer interpreters for languages commonly spoken in the community are available. The effects of medications or phases of illness that temporarily affect mental capabilities can be difficult to recognize and can limit the patient's ability to understand and communicate. Physicians should be encouraged to remove such barriers to decision-making capacity, when medically possible.

Minors and Persons under Guardianship

Although minors and persons under guardianship lack the legal presumption of competency, they should be encouraged to participate in decision making about their own care in ways that are appropriate to their capabilities and maturity. Some minors who have had a chronic disease for a long time, for example, often have substantial insights into the effects and desirability of various alternate courses of treatment. In addition, involving minors in decision making may increase their cooperation with the treatment regimen. Parents or guardians with legal authority to act on the minor's behalf should be encouraged to involve the child appropriately.

State laws sometimes grant minors treatment rights apart from parents in areas such as pregnancy, contraception, abortion, sexually transmitted diseases, and substance abuse. In addition, in some states, minors are considered to be emancipated if they are married or live apart from their parents. Caregivers should be familiar with relevant statutes in their state.

Advance Directives

Advance directives should be considered in the broader context of planning for health care needs. With the increasing prevalence of chronic illness and treatments that are only partially effective, the need for many types of decisions about future health care treatment can be readily anticipated.

An advance directive allows an individual to indicate treatment preferences (often about life-sustaining care) and/or to designate a surrogate decision maker in the event he or she should lack decision-making capacity. An advance directive may be written or oral.

Many states have made statutory provision for two types of advance directive documents: the health care power of attorney (or health care proxy) and the living will (sometimes called natural death declarations). These state laws provide legal protection for health care providers who follow the instructions in a properly prepared document. Health care powers of attorney or health care proxies specify who can make decisions if the patient is unable to do so for himself or herself and may also provide treatment instructions. Living wills give directions to health care providers, often about restricting life-sustaining treatment when death is imminent or unconsciousness is permanent.

It is becoming increasingly common to combine the health care proxy and the living will in one document. The health care proxy is usually considered more flexible, because it applies whenever the patient cannot express himself or herself and allows a surrogate to make decisions on the incapacitated patient's behalf even in circumstances that the patient did not anticipate when preparing the written instruction. Living will documents are often restricted to terminal illness or permanent unconsciousness*, although they may provide guidance on the patient's likely wishes or preferences under other circumstances.

*Consult with legal counsel concerning provisions of state law.

Physicians should be encouraged to discuss the need for advance directives with patients and to talk about the specifics of advance directives with those who have executed them. Studies have shown that individuals with advance directives frequently have not discussed them with their physicians, who, therefore, have no knowledge of them. Also, because the language in many advance directives may be medically vague and subject to many interpretations, physicians should be urged to discuss them with patients. Terms such as *no reasonable expectation of recovery, heroic measures,* or *life-prolonging procedures* are frequently understood differently by different individuals. Any qualifications or restrictions need special attention.

It is common to think of an advance directive as a form, and, indeed, laws in some states require specific forms or language. Many state statutes do not require use of a specific form but do impose certain requirements, such as witnessing, for the statutory immunity provisions to apply. Advance directives that are not on state forms may be written or oral and may convey information concerning values and preferences not accommodated by the statutory form. An advance directive that gives directions that go beyond state law or that fails to satisfy statutory witnessing or documentation requirements nonetheless should serve as guidance and be considered a memorialization of the patient's treatment preferences. In some cases, the hospital may wish to consult an attorney with expertise in the state's laws regarding advance directives, refusal of treatment, and surrogate decision making.

Although living will laws were initially developed to simplify refusal of life-sustaining treatment, some documents or surrogates may ask that everything be done to prolong life. Such requests have implications for resource allocation decisions within the hospital and may also create conflicts for physicians and nurses. A physician who knows or anticipates that this type of request is part of an advance directive should discuss the content in advance with the patient. If the patient is incapacitated and if continued treatment appears to offer no benefit or if treatment is overly burdensome and provides benefits that are at best marginal, such requests should signal the need for discussion with the surrogate. It is usually appropriate for the physician to meet with the surrogate and the patient's family to explain the patient's current status and prognosis and reasons for limiting some kinds of treatment. It may be helpful to include a chaplain, social worker, patient representative, or nurse in these discussions. Consultation with an ethics committee or ethics consultant also may be valuable. Institutions should develop guidelines to address such situations.

Documenting Advance Directives

Advance directives should be documented in or be part of the medical record to ensure that physicians, nurses, and other caregivers have access to them and are better able to provide care consistent with the patient's wishes. Hospitals should have a clear and effective process for obtaining advance directive documents and making them part of the medical record. The written document can be solicited before admission (as part of a preadmission process), at admission, or by securing it from the patient or family during the hospital stay. Health care institutions can ensure that advance directives are carried forward from admission to admission and across institutional settings as appropriate.

If an advance directive document has been developed but cannot be located, the patient should be encouraged to develop a new one. If the patient lacks decision-making capacity, the hospital should have a process by which a social worker, patient representative, member of the clergy, physician, nurse, or other appropriate health care professional talks with the patient's family and other loved ones to try to determine the contents of the advance directive. Substantial effort should be made to ensure that the treatment plan respects the patient's wishes insofar as they are known.

A patient can revoke or change an advance directive at any time in accordance with state laws. Oral expressions by the patient to the physician or others generally have priority over any earlier statement, either oral or written. Hospitals must establish a procedure to document and communicate the change and evaluate the effect of the change on treatment plans. These discussions with the patient and any oral expression of treatment choices should be reflected in the patient's medical record.

Health care decisions are always affected by the context in which they are made, and the patient's general health, medical procedures involved, and prognosis might all affect the patient's choice of treatment. To fully integrate advance directives into hospital care, hospitals should encourage and facilitate patient (or surrogate) review of advance directives, particularly during the admissions process or at the patient's request. Any changes should be reflected in the medical record.

Patient Self-Determination Act

In 1990, Congress passed the Patient Self-Determination Act (PSDA) as part of the Omnibus Budget Reconciliation Act. The purpose of the PSDA is to increase public awareness of advance directives. Each state is required by the PSDA to develop a description of that state's law on advance directives.

The PSDA requires hospitals, nursing homes, home health agencies, HMOs, and other specified providers participating in Medicare and/or Medicaid to:

- Inform adult patients of their rights to make decisions concerning their medical care, including the right to have an advance directive.
- Provide each adult patient with the written policies of the organization with respect to carrying out advance directives.
- Document in the medical record whether the patient has an advance directive.
- Educate staff, physicians, and the community on issues concerning advance directives.

In many cases, individuals choose not to develop an advance directive. The PSDA prohibits any discrimination based on whether a patient has an advance directive.

Patient Preparation of Advance Directives

The Patient Self-Determination Act does not require hospitals to help patients prepare advance directives. However, hospitals are important educational resources in their community with a stake in high-quality health services, and should facilitate preparation of advance directives by patients and community members. Besides physicians, the health care professionals most often involved in helping discuss advance directives are social workers, nurses, patient representatives, and chaplains. Health care institutions should educate staff about how to help patients to develop advance directives without providing legal advice. Institutions should be particularly aware of any state restrictions on whether employees and physicians can witness advance directives or be named as surrogates.

If an institution is unable to provide assistance to patients in preparing advance directives, it should be prepared to refer them to an outside resource.

Surrogate Decision Making

A number of states have adopted health care surrogacy laws, which, in the absence of contrary instructions from the patient, delineate in a specified order those individuals who may make decisions on behalf of a patient when the patient is unable to communicate for himself or herself. Other states have indicated in their summaries of state law prepared in response to the Patient Self-Determination Act that, when there is no patient-designated surrogate, family members are considered appropriate surrogates.

When decisions regarding treatment of an incapacitated patient must be made and no useful guidance concerning designation of an appropriate surrogate is available from the patient or state law, the physician or other caregiver must identify an appropriate surrogate. In these cases, the surrogate should be the person who is likely to know and be willing to assert the patient's values and wishes about treatment, and when these are unknown, who can best represent the patient's best interests.

Often the choice of appropriate surrogate is obvious. The involvement throughout treatment of a spouse, another close relative, or close friend often makes him or her the logical surrogate. Sometimes, there may be multiple surrogates who reach a consensus among themselves and speak on the patient's behalf.

Although state requirements vary greatly, it is usually not necessary to seek court appointment of a legal guardian to identify an appropriate surrogate. When it is difficult to determine the need for or to identify a surrogate decision maker, frequently a hospital ethics committee or ethics consultant can provide additional guidance. The ethical imperative is protection of the patient's interests. Circumstances likely to be most challenging are when:

- The patient's incapacity is great and likely to be prolonged, and there is no obvious surrogate.
- The capacity of the patient is questionable, and the decision to be made is significant.
- The views of the surrogate are strongly at variance with medical judgment or the patient's known views.
- The choice of the individual to serve as surrogate is controversial.
- Family members intractably disagree about the course of action for a patient who is unable to participate in decision making.

If a period of incapacity is likely to result from an illness, treatment, or procedure, the attending physician should encourage the patient to discuss his or her treatment preferences and preferred surrogate in advance. The results of such discussions should be indicated in the patient's records.

The physician and other members of the health care team should work with the surrogate to determine the patient's preferences about health care decisions. Information from living wills, durable powers of attorney for health care, oral communications, other advance directives, and life-style commitments and preferences may provide information about what the patient would have decided under the circumstances. The physician, the health care team, and the family and friends should communicate and work together to make decisions that are consistent with the patient's known views or, if they are not known, with the patient's apparent best interests.

Hospitals should have mechanisms or policies to guide caregivers who believe that a health care surrogate is acting from suspect motives rather than acting consistently with the desires of the patient or in the patient's best interests. If there is some question concerning the appropriateness or legitimacy of the health care surrogate's decision, the responsible health care providers, usually after consultation with an attorney, should determine if the decision or the authority of the surrogate should be contested.

Policies Concerning Life-Sustaining Treatment

Health care institutions should have policies regarding life-sustaining treatment, including resuscitation services. (Specific issues relating to resuscitation services and do-not-resuscitate orders are covered on pages 24.) By developing effective policies in these areas and educating caregivers about their interpretation and application, the hospital is preparing in advance for important—and sometimes controversial—decision making.

These decisions are frequently complicated by the fact that:

- Few patients, while still well, discuss their wishes concerning the circumstances under which they would not want such treatment.
- Physicians may be reluctant to raise the topic with patients.
- The wishes of a patient or family/surrogate may be disregarded because physicians or nurses are concerned about liability or because their values conflict with those of the patient or family/surrogate.
- Specialized legal advice may not be available when needed.

The primary objective of these policies should be to best serve the patient. These policies also serve to:

- Protect patients and families from arbitrarily imposed decisions.
- Guide professionals and institutions in resolving ethical conflicts.
- Help shield the hospital from legal liability or community censure for decisions that are made in good faith.

The Joint Commission on Accreditation of Healthcare Organizations requires policies on withholding and withdrawing life-sustaining treatment, including use and withholding of resuscitation attempts. Although not all hospitals are accredited, JCAHO's requirements are frequently considered to represent recognized standards of practice and so may be relevant to institutions not seeking accreditation. The JCAHO standards attempt to ensure that health care institutions have the functional and structural components necessary for effective policies in place. The Joint Commission's *Accreditation Manual for Hospitals 1994* includes the following relevant standards:

- There are hospitalwide policies on the withholding of resuscitative services from patients and the forgoing or withdrawing of life-sustaining treatment.
- The policies are developed in consultation with the medical staff, nursing staff, and other appropriate bodies and are adopted by the medical staff and approved by the governing body.
- The policies describe:
    - The mechanism(s) for reaching decisions about withholding of resuscitative services from individual patients or forgoing or withdrawing of life-sustaining treatment;
    - The mechanism(s) for resolving conflicts in the decision-making process should they arise; and
    - The roles of physicians and, when applicable, of nursing personnel, other appropriate staff, and family members in the decision to withhold resuscitative services or forgo or withdraw life-sustaining treatment.
- The policies include provisions designed to ensure that patients' rights are respected.
- The policies include the requirement that appropriate orders be written by the physician primarily responsible for the patient's care management and that documentation be made in the patient's medical record if life-

sustaining treatment is to be withdrawn or resuscitative services are to be withheld.

- The policies address the use of advance directives in patient care to the extent permitted by law.

Development of Policies

Although the Joint Commission standards require that these policies be developed in consultation with the medical staff, nursing staff, and other appropriate bodies, development of policies that are useful and functional within the institution requires broader involvement. If feasible, the institution should involve a number of different groups in developing these policies and guidelines and designing educational programs for ensuring appropriate implementation in the institution. These efforts should include representatives from a number of groups within the hospital, including administrators, trustees, medical staff, nursing staff, social workers, pastoral care personnel, and house staff in teaching hospitals. Legal counsel should be available for consultation throughout the process. Health care professionals in different disciplines who have frequent contact with the patient or the patient's family are likely to be aware of a range of issues, concerns, and problems that they encounter in the course of their own work. If the institution has a broadly constituted ethics committee, that committee might well be appropriate for developing or revising such guidelines.

Communication of Treatment Decisions. After decisions have been arrived at by appropriate discussion with patients or surrogates, they must be communicated to all involved health professionals. Policies should stress the importance of discussion as well as written communication. Although much of the rationale should be available in written form, whenever possible the attending physician should discuss the decision with the primary nurse or the nurses who have most contact with the patient. In teaching hospitals, house staff should have the opportunity to discuss the order with the attending physician. Frequently, responses to questions and concerns can minimize conflicts and help caregivers feel more comfortable with particular decisions. In the case of DNR orders, it is particularly critical that policies emphasize that the decision to rescind a DNR order is communicated to all caregivers who are aware of the previous DNR order but might not have been on duty when the decision was made to rescind it.

Policies should delineate the physician's responsibilities for discussing these treatment issues with the patient, the patient's surrogate, or the patient's family. When needed, the physician should help the designated surrogate discuss the issues with the patient's family. Most institutional policies require consent for a DNR order; however, each institution should exercise discretion in determining whether consent is needed for all DNR orders, particularly in cases where attempts at resuscitation are reliably expected to fail.

Legal Issues and Conflicts. Relevant state statutes or case law, such as those regarding DNR orders, termination of life-sustaining treatment, living wills, and durable powers of attorney for health care, should be taken into account in the development of policies. In addition, policies should identify situations in which additional legal guidance may be needed, such as the case of an emancipated minor or confusion concerning the appropriate surrogate decision maker.

Policies should recognize that at times there will not be complete agreement. Conflicts can result from differences in medical judgments as well as differences in values. They can occur between an attending physician and another health care professional, between an attending physician and a consulting physician, between an attending physician and the patient or the patient's family, between the patient and the patient's family, or among family members. Clearly, it is in the best interest of all to resolve these conflicts as fairly and expeditiously as possible.

When there is uncertainty about the medical status of the patient and whether a patient would be well served by life-sustaining treatment and/or attempts at resuscitation, the policy should encourage physicians to seek medical consultation with other physicians or, in some cases, the hospital ethics committee. The medical record should reflect other professional consultations, if any.

Policies should discuss various conflict resolution steps and options, including possible recourse to the courts, depending on the type of conflict. Decisions should be made at the closest possible level to the patient, taking into account the therapeutic relationship between patient and caregivers, patient privacy, and the possibility that court proceedings may be costly and may involve judges who lack expertise in the area of law and medicine. Although recourse to the court system should rarely be needed, when it is appropriate, a court decision should be sought promptly, with the right information, and without rancor.

Effective conflict resolution steps can include clinical consultation in the case of disagreement about a medical condition, and consultation with pastoral staff, an ethics consultant (if such a service is available at the institution), or an ethics committee. At times, allowing a caregiver to transfer to a different unit or ensuring that caregivers are not responsible for carrying out an order to which they object on the basis of personal beliefs can effectively address the problem.

Policies on resuscitation and withdrawing or withholding of life-sustaining treatment obviously cannot ensure that all caregivers in the hospital have a shared belief or value structure. They should, however, define the bases for making and implementing these decisions.

Review of Policies. Before a final policy or policy revision is approved, it is important that a draft be widely circulated for review within the institution to ensure that it provides adequate support and direction for making and implementing these decisions. Chiefs of clinical services, chief residents, clinical nurse managers, ethics committee members, and directors of social work, pastoral care, and patient representative services should generally have an opportunity to comment on the draft. Legal review is also needed. Although this review process may seem cumbersome, it can help identify important omissions or implementation problems in the policy. In addition, being given an opportunity to comment and suggest changes gives caregivers a vested interest in making the policy work.

As with all policies, the hospital should regularly review and evaluate its experience with these decisions and orders and their implementation.

Issues for Special Consideration

Withdrawing vs. Withholding Treatment. At times, health care professionals or family members may feel more uncomfortable about the prospect of withdrawing life-sustaining treatment than they do about withholding that treatment entirely. There is discomfort with the notion of *taking something away* once it has been started. It may seem more *active* than the more passive act of withholding. State laws and court opinions have determined, however, that there is no decisive difference between withdrawing and withholding treatment. In a few states, specific procedures are specified that differ for withdrawing or withholding. Many health care professionals point out that if criteria for withdrawing treatment are more stringent than for withholding treatment, there may be a strong disincentive to going forward with a *trial of treatment*—to the detriment of patient care. A time-limited *trial of treatment* frequently can help to determine more clearly diagnosis, prognosis, and optimal treatment. Such issues should be addressed in the relevant policies.

Nutrition and Hydration. Appellate court cases have affirmed that artificial nutrition and hydration are considered to be forms of treatment that may be withheld or withdrawn, under appropriate circumstances. Under some state advance directive statutes, unless individuals indicate specifically in their formal advance directives that they would want artificial nutrition and hydration withheld or withdrawn, those treatments may not be withheld. The constitutionality and enforceability of these statutes are uncertain. Some institutions—for religious or other reasons—will develop policies refusing to withhold or withdraw articifial nutrition or hydration. These policies must be clearly stated and made well-known to patients, and institutions should develop procedures for transferring patients or making other appropriate arrangements when such requests are made.

Futility. Much health care emphasizes curing and rehabilitative care, which attempts to restore the patient to health, or, when that is not possible, to cure a specific medical problem. Increasingly, as the population ages, life spans lengthen, and partially effective treatment becomes more common, caregivers and patients alike are reconsidering the wisdom of burdensome treatment that will not ultimately serve the patient's interest. Invasive or burdensome treatment frequently is not appropriate for patients with chronic disease and multiple debilitating conditions. In cases where a patient has many serious medical problems, effective treatment for one condition may not be expected to contribute to his or her general well-being or to a positive outcome, as defined by the patient. Treatment in such cases is frequently described as *futile*.

The meaning and usefulness of the term *futility* are under debate in the academic and scholarly literature. The term, nonetheless, is frequently used and heard in the health care setting. Some restrict the definition of futility to treatment having no beneficial physiological effect. Others attempt to define futility by reference to statistical data on the likelihood of success— a treatment that does not reach a particular statistical threshold is considered futile. Others look at the treatment's effect on the quality of life—even if a treatment is successful, it would not raise the patient's quality of life to an acceptable state, as defined by the patient. Still others label futile treatment that seems to cause more suffering and harm than good. When caregivers believe that instead of caring for a patient they are inflicting unnecessary pain, they commonly attribute their anguish to the *futility* of what they are being asked to do.

Some have argued that interventions physicians deem futile need not be offered or discussed or may be withheld or withdrawn without patient or surrogate consent. In view of the controversy over defining futile treatment, this approach risks denying important patient and family rights. A better approach would be for health care institutions and networks to help create an environment where caregivers can provide better information to families and can better communicate their discomfort with treatment, both among themselves and with the patient or the patient's surrogate/family. Surrogates or family members may be unaware of the pain or trauma to patients associated with some treatments. Forthright discussion may yield different, and better, decisions on treatment. Nevertheless, there is some point at which a treatment is either so unlikely to work or so unlikely to benefit the patient's life that professional standards should allow the treatment not to be offered.

Palliative Care and Pain Management. A decision to refuse or cease one kind of treatment does not mean that the patient no longer receives care. The emphasis often shifts from correcting physiological abnormalities to determining how to best provide palliative care and keep the patient comfortable. Questions as to what treatment and how much medication or sedation are appropriate should reflect the needs and values of each individual patient. The greatest fear of some patients may be unremitting pain; for others, it may be the inability to think clearly and communicate. Appropriate medication for one may be inappropriate for another.

Physicians sometimes hesitate to prescribe effective pain medication because, while relieving symptoms and pain, the medication may also slow respiratory functions or, in other ways, hasten death. Effective pain management may also be hindered because of concerns about addiction, even in terminally ill patients. Neither concern is an appropriate barrier to fully effective pain relief when that is what serves the patient best.

Policies of health care networks and hospitals should recognize that effective pain management is necessary both within and outside the acute care setting. When possible, hospitals and networks should make available formal or informal pain consultation services to help physicians manage pain appropriately. Formularies should ensure that appropriate pain-relieving pharmaceuticals are available to physicians. In-service education programs should be developed to educate physicians and other caregivers about the ethics of and need for pain management as well as dispel myths and fears surrounding it. Caregivers must understand that a patient's decision to forgo life-sustaining treatment does not mean the end of providing care. It signals the need to redouble efforts to provide palliation and pain relief. Often, physical suffering is accompanied by emotional pain, and caregivers, including nurses, social workers, and chaplains, can help ease the patient's pain through listening, empathizing, and counseling.

DNR Orders

At various times during the course of a patient's illness, the patient, the patient's surrogate, the family, and caregivers will need to discuss whether cardiopulmonary resuscitation (CPR) should be attempted if the patient's heart stops. CPR is a procedure of artificial respiration and manual external cardiac massage. A defibrillator and various drugs are also used to restore a heartbeat.

The patient's preferences and the expected outcome of resuscitation should determine resuscitation status. If resuscitation has a reasonable chance of success and the patient has indicated that the quality of life before or after resuscitation is or would be acceptable, then a do-not-resuscitate (DNR) order is not warranted. It should be clear to all caregivers that a DNR order can be compatible with full therapeutic treatment, although at times it may be combined with orders for palliative or comfort treatment.

The need for a DNR order should be considered independently from advance directives. An advance directive may indicate the circumstances under which a DNR order should be written for an incapacitated patient. However, DNR orders may also be appropriate where there are no advance directives.

Generally, there are three distinct justifications for DNR orders:

- There is no medical benefit to treatment. Attempted resuscitation would be futile in that it cannot be expected to restore circulation.
- The quality of life after resuscitation would be less desirable to the patient than death resulting from a cardiac arrest. The patient's life would be so marked by suffering or so limited in its opportunities that the patient would prefer not to have survived. An example would be a cardiac patient whose brain had become severely damaged because of an arrest and for whom resuscitation efforts had caused permanent ventilator dependency.
- The quality of life before resuscitation is such that the patient would prefer death resulting from a cardiac arrest. In such cases (e.g., a person in a persistent vegetative state or with disabling and painful end-stage cancer), a successful resuscitation is viewed by the patient (or the patient's family and physician) as having no benefit, because the net burden of life was already considered less desirable than death from a cardiac arrest.

Slow Codes and Partial Codes. Because it creates a false impression of fully attempting resuscitation, a slow code is not an ethical alternative to the DNR order. It is not an acceptable method of avoiding difficult discussions with the patient or the patient's family or for resolving conflicts between the patient's family and the caregivers on the appropriateness of DNR orders. In addition, slow codes are subject to broad interpretation and cause difficult dilemmas for caregivers.

Partial codes are sometimes viewed differently from slow codes. Partial codes may include DNR orders with additional instructions to initiate only specific parts of CPR. Although allowing patients and surrogates to request only some parts of resuscitation maximizes patient autonomy, given the low rate of success of resuscitation, limiting use of some valuable components makes success virtually unattainable.

Under no circumstances should a partial code be used in place of a DNR order to accommodate poor communication among caregivers and patients and families/surrogates. Patients and surrogates should be told of the implication of a partial code for successful resuscitation. If a partial code is deemed acceptable, it is imperative that all language be well-defined, that specific elements included be documented, and that written unambiguous instructions anticipate possible medical interventions.

DNR Policy Issues. Although policies regarding DNR orders and withholding/withdrawal of life-sustaining treatment may be similar in many respects, policies on DNR orders should give particular attention to how to address issues that frequently arise in relation to DNR policies and orders. These include the following:

- Attending physicians may be reluctant to initiate discussions about DNR orders with patients.
- The circumstances under which a DNR order would be appropriate may not be considered until a crisis develops, when it may be too late to speak with family members or medical consultants.
- Conflicts about interpretation of a DNR order may arise among medical staff or between physicians and nurses.
- Patients with DNR orders may receive a different standard of care than other patients, because staff may assume that treatment in addition to resuscitation attempts is not desired or, alternatively, fear of substandard care may prevent patients or families/surrogates from considering DNR orders.

Some of these problems can be minimized with revision or better drafting of DNR policies. Others require better implementation of orders. Still others must be addressed by staff and patient education. To ensure that a policy on DNR orders is understood and uniformly implemented throughout the hospital, the policy should:

- Clearly define critical terms, including do-not-resuscitate, cardiopulmonary resuscitation, and any additional terms that are subject to differing interpretations.
- Specify what terminology should be used in authorizing DNR orders and where such orders should be recorded.
- Indicate appropriate confirmation of orders that have been communicated over a facsimile machine, telephone, computer, or other electronic device.
- Address the validity of existing DNR orders for patients transferred to the hospital and indicate how long a previous order may be in effect prior to reassessment.
- Specify where and how the relevant discussions about the DNR order should be recorded so that nursing, house staff, and others involved in the patient's care have ready access to information explaining who was involved in the decision, what assumptions were made, and under what type of circumstances the DNR order should be reevaluated.
- Emphasize that the patient's attending physician is responsible for the decision to authorize a DNR order and specify what circumstances would justify a different physician making such a decision.
- Address who is responsible for authorizing and writing DNR orders for emergency room patients and recognize that different procedures may be needed for emergency room patients with physicians on staff but not present at the hospital than for emergency room patients without a physician on staff at the institution.
- Specify the minimum frequency with which a decision related to resuscitation should be evaluated and make it clear that review is required whenever a patient's medical status changes in an unexpected manner or worsens, or when an active medical intervention that poses risk of an iatrogenic arrest is required.
- Indicate the attending physician is primarily responsible for reviewing the order, but nursing staff and other caregivers, who may have more frequent contact with the patient, have a responsibility for informing the physician about changes in condition that call for reconsideration of a decision for CPR or a DNR order.
- Specify the appropriate physician to authorize or rescind a DNR order.
- Emphasize respect and concern for the patient's wishes by promoting early discussion, clear communication, and accurate record keeping.

Patient Care Environment

The previous chapter, **Making Patient Care Decisions**, stressed the need for health care policies to ensure a supportive and collaborative environment for making treatment decisions. The overall patient care environment must also respect and support patient dignity and autonomy in the context of a health care system that serves the community, provides needed care for all people, and stresses high-quality patient care outcomes. This responsibility begins with the governing body of the institution or network and should become a part of the culture of the entire organization, including medical staff, caregivers, and support and administrative staff.

The AHA's *A Patient's Bill of Rights* (Appendix B) sets forth 12 patient rights and calls on hospitals to:

. . .provide a foundation for understanding and respecting the rights and responsibilities of patients, their families, physicians, and other caregivers. . .ensure a health care ethic that respects the role of patients in decision making about treatment choices and other aspects of care. . .be sensitive to cultural, racial, linguistic, religious, age, gender, and other differences as well as the needs of persons with disabilities.

The patient care environment is shaped by many issues, some almost intangible—such as the thoughtfulness and openness of caregivers and other personnel—and others that are more amenable to development of policy and evaluation. The latter include how providers address competency and quality of care issues, the extent to which confidentiality of patient information is stressed, how conflicts are handled, how restraints are used, and how professional and moral values of caregivers are respected.

Competency and Quality of Care

The hospital has an ethical and legal responsibility to make certain that the health care provided by its employees and by physicians and others with hospital privileges meets acceptable standards. Hospitals should ensure that all those providing patient care are appropriately educated, trained, and currently competent. Each institution should have a rigorous procedure for verifying credentials of applicants for medical staff membership and clinical privileges, as well as of medical students and residents, nurses, therapists, and other health care professionals. Federal law requires hospitals to query the National Practitioner Data Bank for information on adverse licensure actions, adverse clinical privilege actions, and medical malpractice payment information on physicians when they initially apply for medical staff membership and every two years thereafter for each physician holding medical staff membership and clinical privileges.

Disclosing Adverse Events

The way a hospital deals with unplanned outcomes and errors in care has significant ramifications for its ethical relationships with its patients and community.

Unplanned Outcomes. The hospital should have a procedure for informing patients in advance about possible unplanned, but statistically possible, outcomes, such as nosocomial infections or side effects of treatment regimens, as well as a procedure for informing the patient if an unplanned outcome does occur.

Errors. If a treatment error occurs, the hospital has a strong duty of prompt and full disclosure to the patient or surrogate. Hospitals and health care professionals must acknowledge that some errors are inevitable and may occur under conditions ordinarily associated with good results. Such acknowledgment is an important element of professionalism and conducive to the sharing of information and reducing error to a minimum. The institution should create an environment in which health care professionals are encouraged to report adverse outcomes.

Disclosure Procedures. Institutions should have a written policy on disclosure of errors to patients and families, including the appropriate format of such disclosure, the appropriate timing of the disclosure, what is to be disclosed, and to whom information is to be disclosed. The hospital attorney should be involved in drafting the policy, and the policy should indicate when legal counsel involvement and/or notification is needed. Full disclosure of significant errors is based on the patient's right to know and should be supported even in cases where the error has been corrected and the patient is no longer harmed. This approach may need to acknowledge that the disclosure of an already-ameliorated error may be distressing to the patient.

Ordinarily, the professional involved in the error should be involved in the disclosure to the patient, and available information should be fully disclosed to the patient or the patient's surrogate. Timely disclosure to and prompt communication with patients and their families can greatly mitigate the impact of an adverse event. Disclosure also should include what happened; the causes, if known; and any known effects on the patient's short-term and long-term health. Disclosures should include treatment options to overcome or compensate for the effects of the error on the patient.

Partial disclosure—either stemming from risk management concerns or physician or hospital judgments of patient interest—restricts the patient's autonomy and requires appropriate consultation and discussion by the health care team; it should not be decided unilaterally by the individual who made the error. A position that partial or nondisclosure serves the patient's well-being requires careful scrutiny to determine if it could be a response to a conflict of interest. Delays or cover-ups are neither morally nor legally acceptable alternatives; they violate respect for the patient and often increase the liability exposure of institutions and individuals involved.

Hospital policy should assist health care administrators and clinical caregivers to distinguish between significant and insignificant errors in patient care and respond appropriately. Insignificant errors may require only an incident report. For example, administering a medication an hour late may have no appreciable effect on the patient. A more significant accident or oversight that may result in significant short- or long-term harm to a patient requires positive action and full disclosure.

Reporting to Authorities

In some cases, hospitals and health care professionals are legally required to report to appropriate professional and/or federal or state authorities unsafe or unethical practices, particularly those that have not been eliminated or corrected through earlier efforts.

Some adverse outcomes must be reported under the Safe Medical Devices Act of 1990, which requires user facilities, including hospitals, to report to the Food and Drug Administration or the manufacturer when it *receives or otherwise becomes aware of information that reasonably suggests that there is a probability that a device has caused or contributed to* the death, serious illness, or serious injury of a patient of the facility. Also, hospitals must report to the National Practitioner Data Bank information on adverse actions on clinical privileges such as suspension for 30 days or longer or payments made for the benefit of physicians, dentists, and other health care practitioners as a result of medical malpractice actions and claims.

Handling Potentially Impaired Medical and Hospital Staff

Substance abuse, infectious disease, dementia, and other problems may at times interfere with the ability of health care professionals to carry out their duties with consequences for quality of health care. Hospitals should have procedures for identifying and dealing with such impairments, while protecting the staff member's confidentiality.

Hospitals should adopt a rehabilitative or therapeutic approach to substance abuse in the workplace, focusing on referral to internal or external employee assistance programs or professional treatment to assist employees or medical staff members willing to recognize and overcome their substance abuse. Although disciplinary measures, such as suspension, reassignment of duties, or restricted access to medications, may be necessary in some cases, health care institutions should emphasize rehabilitation, and employees and medical staff members who successfully complete treatment should be provided with an opportunity to continue working in the institution.

Health care workers infected with HIV or HBV (hepatitis B) do not need to be removed from patient care duties if they are otherwise capable of performing their tasks and adequate precautions to protect both health care workers and patients can be taken. Decisions on what tasks an HIV-infected health care worker can perform should take into account both physical and mental effects of the disease process and the theoretical risk of transmission to patients and other health care workers. For HBV, risks are small but greater than for HIV. Institutions should determine fitness for duty for HIV-infected and HBV-infected health care workers on a case-by-case basis. Hospitals should establish mechanisms within their existing worker impairment programs to determine whether a health care worker known to be infected with HIV or HBV can adequately and safely perform patient care duties.

Monitoring and Improving System Performance

Hospitals and health care networks must continue to monitor and work to improve health care quality. Tissue committees, quality management programs, review of credentials, and utilization review all play a role in detecting problems related to the competency of various health care professionals. Increasingly, collection and dissemination of statistical information on the quality of care is being used to monitor care and to provide accountability to the community. In addition, meaningful information can help people choose among providers, practitioners, and networks. Care should be taken to ensure that data on quality and patterns of care are relevant and are used appropriately. Providers and practitioners should collaborate on producing and integrating data about quality of care. For example, information on patterns of practice and patient outcome could be compiled across hospitals or by integrating information from physicians, hospitals, nursing facilities, and other providers and practitioners.

Implementing a Reporting Mechanism

Beyond these efforts, hospitals and health networks should create an environment that provides maximum protection for patients from incompetent, illegal, or unethical practices. This concern extends to all patient care activities, whether conducted by an independent physician, a physician employed by or under contract to the hospital, another hospital employee, or a volunteer. Hospitals and networks should encourage their medical staffs, employees, and volunteers to recognize when the patient care practices of others present a danger to the health or safety of patients and to make certain that appropriate steps are taken to rectify the problem. They should have clearly defined, publicized, and easily accessible mechanisms for receiving, investigating, and taking action on disclosures and allegations of unethical behavior or incompetence by health care professionals. These mechanisms will vary depending on organizational structure and size, but it should be remembered that direct reporting of such problems to supervisors may be unrealistic in some cases and alternatives provided. The chosen system should protect the rights of all parties—the individuals who disclose information, the involved health care professionals, and the patient.

Hospitals and health networks should have mechanisms to ensure that patients have an established and publicized method of voicing concern about what they perceive to be unsafe or unethical practices. Patient information materials should identify who should be contacted with concerns about care. Patient representatives, ombudsmen, social workers, chaplains, or administrators may all be appropriate contacts for patients. Although some patient concerns may be based on a lack of understanding of medical procedures and hospital routines, the observations may help identify patterns of questionable care. Patient reporting of concerns gives health care professionals an opportunity to correct problems as well as to explain procedures that may be misunderstood by or disturbing to patients.

Creating an atmosphere conducive to prompt and appropriate disclosure puts the network, the hospital, and caregivers on record as not tolerating practices and continued performance that are below standard. To achieve this perspective, efforts must be thorough and confidential, and provide responsive, timely investigation and corrective action.

Confidentiality

Patients have the right to expect that all communication and records pertaining to their care will be treated as confidential by the hospital and health care network. Since the earliest practice of medicine, the confidentiality of patient information has been a foremost tenet. Despite this long tradition of confidentiality, changes in the environment of the hospital, laws and regulations, and activities of third-party payers are affecting the range and type of information deemed confidential.

The American Hospital Association's *A Patient's Bill of Rights* sums up confidentiality from the patient's perspective:

The patient has the right to every consideration of privacy. Case discussion, consultation, examination, and treatment should be conducted so as to protect each patient's privacy. ...The patient has the right to expect that all communications and records pertaining to his/her care will be treated as confidential by the hospital, except in cases such as suspected abuse and public health hazards when reporting is permitted or required by law. The patient has the right to expect that the hospital will emphasize the confidentiality of this information when it releases it to any other parties entitled to review information in these records.

Values in Conflict

In the age of computers at the bed side, nursing stations, laboratories, and physician offices, opportunities increasingly exist to gain access to patient information. As integrated medical records develop more fully and begin to follow patients throughout their health care system contacts, more and more people will come into contact with sensitive patient information. Some will have legitimate need for the information. Confidential patient information may be needed by payers, peer review committees, and the various caregivers, specialists, and consultants who see a particular patient. Although current laws on protecting the confidentiality of individually identifiable health care information vary by state, many health care leaders (including the American Hospital Association) have called for national standards.

Hospitals and health care networks have a legal and moral responsibility to establish institutional mechanisms and practices to protect the confidentiality of patient information and limit access to patient records to appropriate individuals.

Because patients must share information about personal habits, history, and circumstances relevant to their health or illness with physicians and other health care professionals, the hospital must develop policies that protect and support a climate conducive to confidentiality and clarify when strict confidentiality may be overridden. Hospitals should develop clear rules authorizing access to information and clear disciplinary procedures and sanctions for those breaching confidentiality. Certain information about patients, such as substance abuse, HIV infection, psychiatric illness, or reproductive history, is particularly sensitive, and hospitals should enforce strict adherence to the principle of confidentiality. Issues such as the use of patient information in education and research should be considered, and policy should stress that the duty of confidentiality is not a function of the source of financing of the patient's care.

To help assure a climate of confidentiality, all those in the hospital should be informed of and understand the hospital's practices concerning access to and use of patient information. To enhance this climate, the hospital should actively discourage any discussion of case material in public areas and may wish to establish nonpublic areas specifically for discussion of cases by the health care team.

Patient Consent for Disclosure	The right of the patient to request or sanction disclosure of otherwise confidential personal information takes precedence over the hospital's obligation to protect it. These disclosures can be informal—for example, when physicians or other caregivers provide information to family members. Hospitals should encourage physicians and other caregivers to seek the patient's permission to disclose confidential information to the patient's family whenever possible and, if the physician anticipates the patient will be temporarily unable to communicate, to seek permission in advance.

When patients give consent for the release of their medical records, the hospital should help patients understand their option to limit the scope of the information to be disclosed to the minimum necessary. In signing consents for release of information to insurers and others, patients may not be aware that they may restrict disclosure to specific types of information for specific purposes. When it appropriately discloses information, the hospital should emphasize the information is confidential and the receiving party is required to maintain its confidentiality.

Overriding Confidentiality	Subject to state law, confidentiality may be overridden when the life or safety of the patient is endangered, such as when knowledgeable intervention can prevent threatened suicide or self-injury. In addition, the moral obligation to prevent substantial and foreseeable physical harm to an identifiable third party usually is greater than the moral obligation to protect confidentiality. Protection of the interests or rights of the public as a whole also may override the obligation of confidentiality. Common examples of such overriding interests, as defined by state laws, include child abuse or patients posing a danger to society.

In addition, hospitals, physicians, nurses, and others have legal duties to report certain communicable diseases, injuries, and other conditions to public health officials or other appropriate authorities. Notifying partners of HIV-infected individuals is a controversial issue, with some state laws specifying what disclosure is required, permitted, or prohibited. Notification may help partners to change behavior or to seek early treatment if they have become infected. However, the possibility of partner notification may deter HIV-infected individuals from seeking testing and treatment. While most frequently physicians or public health professionals are likely to be most involved in issues of partner notification, hospitals may wish to have a process to assist HIV-infected individuals in making disclosure to partners.

Institutional Provision of Ethics Committees and Ethics Consultation

Hospital mechanisms for addressing ethical issues and conflicts, such as ethics committees and ethics consultants, are becoming increasingly common, partly as a result of accreditation standards of the Joint Commission on Accreditation of Healthcare Organizations and legislation in some states that require hospitals to have a mechanism for conflict resolution and guidance on ethical issues. As of 1992, more than half of community hospitals reported having an ethics committee. Other parties involved in conflict resolution and guidance include patient representatives, physicians, and pastoral care; formal mechanisms include mediation or other legal and patient services. Each institution needs to determine when an ethics consultant, an ethics committee, or some other approach best meets its needs.

Ethics Committees

Ethics committees are not a recent phenomenon. They have existed under other names in many health care institutions, particularly church-related hospitals, for some time. Yet, today's increasing proliferation of ethics committees, ethics consultations, and other conflict resolution and guidance mechanisms introduces important considerations for what these mechanisms should and should not do, how they should operate, and how they can most successfully carry out their functions. Much has been learned about ethics committees and ethics consultation over the past decade; much useful data still remain to be gathered.

Although conflict resolution and guidance mechanisms such as ethics committees and ethics consultants hold promise for assisting patients, their families, and health care professionals to make decisions well, they should not replace the traditional loci of patient care decision making. Ethics committees should not serve as professional conduct review boards or as substitutes for legal or judicial review. They should also be distinct from institutional review boards, which review clinical research.

Functions. Functions commonly assigned to ethics committees include the following:

- **Serving in an advisory capacity and/or as a resource to persons involved in biomedical decision making.** The use of ethics committees in an advisory role to assist physicians, other health care professionals, and patients and their families who are confronted with dilemmas is probably their most complex function. Ethics committees may make recommendations at the request of an attending physician, nurse, or other hospital professional closely connected with the case, the hospital administration, and the patient or the patient's family. Policies on documenting recommendations in the patient's medical records should be determined by each institution.
- **Retrospectively reviewing decisions having biomedical ethical implications.** Knowledge gained through reviewing past decision-making processes or other ethics-related issues can help guide and improve future decision making.
- **Serving as an institutional resource for development and revision of institutional policies related to bioethical issues.** Such institutional policies can include issues of patient decision making (informed consent, assessment of capacity, role of minors and others without legal capacity), confidentiality, do-not-resuscitate orders, and use of restraints (see related sections).
- **Evaluating compliance with hospital policies related to ethical issues.** Ethics committees may examine compliance with relevant hospital policies such as those related to do-not-resuscitate orders or the Patient Self-Determination Act.
- **Directing educational programs on biomedical ethics issues.** Educational programs on biomedical ethics issues serve to heighten awareness and provide guidance on identification of cases where ethical problems may arise. Such programs may be offered to medical staff, the hospital staff, and the community.
- **Providing forums for discussion among hospital and medical professionals and others about biomedical ethical issues.** Forums for discussion of these issues provide an opportunity for physicians, nurses, administrators, trustees, clergy, ethicists, social workers, and others to consider and discuss a number of diverse perspectives.
- **Networking with other ethics committees.** When there are multiple ethics committees in a community, they may find it productive and efficient to work together to pro-

vide educational programming for the community or develop self-education programs for their own members. Some areas have organized ethics committee networks, which can be found through state and local hospital associations, medical school or university programs in ethics, and ethics publications.

Composition. The members of an ethics committee should be selected in keeping with its objectives and represent a range of perspectives and expertise. It should be multidisciplinary and may include physicians, nurses, administrators, social workers, psychologists, respiratory therapists, clergy, trustees, attorneys, ethicists, and patient advocates (representatives). Community members may be included at the hospital's discretion, with their contributions particularly appropriate on those ethics committees involved in community education. Hospital legal counsel should be available at the request of the committee, and, in some cases, legal review of committee recommendations may be necessary.

To be most useful and effective, an ethics committee should be a standing committee, and its members should be approved by the appropriate authority within the institution. This structure provides continuity and enhances the credibility of the committee. The committee should meet regularly to discuss educational, programmatic, and policy activities and whenever necessary to provide advice and recommendations.

Self-Evaluation. To ensure that ethics committees are functioning appropriately, committees should have a clearly identified purpose, an explicit understanding of their functions, and formal procedures that help accomplish that purpose. Ethics committees should have processes to ensure that important facts in the cases reviewed are available and considered by the committee and that opinions of all committee members are elicited. They should have a written statement of purpose and function and a periodic, formalized evaluation process. The committee's evaluation should include accomplishments, strengths, weaknesses, effectiveness of committee communication with the hospital medical staff and other health care professionals through policies and guidelines, and other pertinent issues. Although self-assessment can be an effective review and learning mechanism for hospital ethics committees, the evaluation of the ethics committee may also be incorporated into other hospital mechanisms ensuring quality of care.

Confidentiality. In the deliberations of ethics committees and ethics consultants, the confidentiality of patient information and the patient's privacy must be respected. All those involved with the ethics committee must be sensitive to the need for confidentiality.

In some hospitals, particularly public institutions, confidentiality is a factor in determining the place of the committee in the hospital structure. For example, if records of administration or governance committees are subject to public disclosure, then establishing an ethics committee as a medical staff committee (with multidisciplinary membership) would better ensure confidentiality.

Consent for Case Review. The hospital should communicate state law and hospital policies regarding use of ethics committees and ethics consultation services in its information materials for patients and families. When committee recommendations may influence decisions on the patient's care or treatment plan, patients or their surrogates should be informed of any impending review and invited to attend some portion of the ethics committee meeting. If the patient or his or her surrogate objects to the review, the review should not proceed. Patients or their surrogates might prefer that the ethics committee not review a case because of privacy concerns (for example, the patient is a hospital employee or otherwise known in the hospital and community) or because of patient or surrogate concerns about potentially coercive powers of the ethics committee decision. Although an ethics committee is only advisory, ethics committee opinions have gained great weight both within hospitals and, increasingly, within some courts.

If a case identifies issues that would be useful for educating or providing general guidance on ethical concerns to physicians and other health care professionals, the ethics committee should seek ways to raise the issues that are separate from case review and do not identify the patient.

Access to Ethics Committee. Everyone involved in the hospital—medical staff, nurses, other employees, trustees, volunteers, patients, and patients' families—should have access to the ethics committee as a resource, and the referral process should be well-publicized. In its advisory capacity, it should be open to those seeking counsel about the range of ethically acceptable responses to a conflict of values.

Ethics Committees and Resource Allocation. Clearly, resource allocation or rationing can raise ethical issues. Some ethics committees have successfully carved out a role beyond acute care and individual patients' treatment plans, for example, urging a greater hospital role in drug treatment. Some hospitals have separate corporate ethics committees dedicated to resource allocation.

Ethics committees can, of course, play an important role in advocating for patient and community needs and can help ensure that all points of view are represented in resource allocation decisions, balancing resource use and benefits. However, taking on the job of helping balance resource use on the institutional level may limit the ethics committee's time and capacity to address direct patient care issues.

Each institution must recognize and balance these trade-offs in deciding whether its ethics committee should become involved in resource allocation decisions.

Hospitals should also recognize that although the patient's financial considerations might be taken into account by an ethics committee in its overall efforts to identify the range of ethically acceptable alternatives in a given situation, financial issues should not be a foremost consideration for case review ethics committees, nor should an ethics committee be asked to play the role of de facto rationer of health care services on a patient-by-patient basis.

Ethics Consultants

Many institutions, particularly university hospitals and other institutions closely affiliated with academic institutions, are increasingly using ethics consultants to assist in resolving patient care ethics dilemmas. Both ethics consultants and ethics committees have their own set of advantages and can be used within the same institution under different circumstances. Ethics consultants offer ease of scheduling a consultation and fewer confidentiality concerns. Ethics committees pool the expertise and perspectives of a number of different individuals from different disciplines.

Restraints on Patients

Restraints include bedside rails, safety vests, waist restraints, wrist restraints, and tranquilizers and other chemical restraints. Patient restraints should be used only when necessary and the restraints chosen should be the least restrictive possible. Use of physical or chemical restraints requires patient or surrogate consent or evidence of a danger posed by the patient to himself or herself or to others. Particular caution should be exercised in using any restraint on a routine basis or by standing order. Because chemical restraints may impair the patient's ability to participate fully in decisions about treatment, their use should be carefully scrutinized. (Also see barriers to capacity on p. 11.)

Confusion and agitation may justify restraints, or they may be aggravated by restraint use. The application of restraints should not serve as a substitute for dealing with confusion and agitation as symptoms of other problems that require medical attention.

Restraints also should not be used for management convenience or to compensate for inadequate staffing patterns, although it should be recognized that some restraint use may be justifiable even with excellent staffing levels.

Because the potential for abuse of restraints extends beyond psychiatric and institutional long-term care, hospital policies should address the ethical use of restraints in all hospital services.

The Joint Commission on Accreditation of Healthcare Organizations' *Accreditation Manual for Hospitals, 1994* requires a hospitalwide policy that specifies the time within which an order must be obtained after each use of restraint or seclusion and the maximum time for the use of either intervention. The JCAHO also requires that the policy address periodic observation of patients for whom restraint or seclusion is employed, including a maximum time between observations.

When developing policies, hospitals should consult with their legal counsel because state laws differ on authorization for restraints.

Although not required directly by the Joint Commission, policies also should provide guidance on the following:

- Authorization of restraints.
- Documentation of the types of behavior justifying use of restraints.

- Appropriate communication with the patient and the patient's family about the need for restraints.
- Documentation of a decision by a patient with adequate decision-making capacity, or a patient's surrogate, regarding use of a restraint.
- Proper fitting of a physical restraint or titration of a chemical restraint to minimize the risk of harm to the patient.

Hospitals should educate staff on alternatives to restraints and encourage them to develop and use alternatives when possible. Particular attention should be paid to the role of the nurse, who is usually the health care professional applying restraints and most affected by their application. Nurses should be encouraged to discuss the use and removal of restraints for particular patients with attending physicians, and hospitals should have procedures to follow when nurses and physicians do not agree on appropriate action and when potential danger to the patient or others is a factor.

Health Care Professionals— Moral Prerogatives and Limits

Although in great part, this report has emphasized the need for a hospital environment conducive to ensuring respect for the patient's self-determination and autonomy, some attention to the moral prerogatives of health care professionals is warranted. Sometimes the patient's or surrogate's treatment choice clashes with caregivers' professional or individual moral values. Hospitals and networks must have policies and procedures to address such conflict.

Institutions have an obligation to try to keep personal objections of caregivers from disrupting care. At the same time, institutions should make reasonable efforts to accommodate health care professionals' personal moral, religious, or cultural values.

Caregivers must inform the hospital or health network of personal moral, religious, or cultural values that may preclude their taking part in certain procedures or withholding or providing certain kinds of care. If these objections fall within legitimate claims of moral prerogatives, the hospital should try to have other personnel available to provide or withhold care as requested. The hospital should not allow the patient's care to be compromised because of internal conflicts of values.

Health care professionals have certain obligations to deliver care, which may be articulated in their professional codes of ethics. Claims of moral prerogatives do not legitimately allow health care professionals to refuse to provide care based on perceptions of the patient's social worth, life-style, or culture.

Clearly, there are no easy answers when health care workers' professional and personal values conflict with patient decisions. Hospitals must be sensitive to these dilemmas and develop appropriate organizational support systems and resolution techniques. Hospitals should be sensitive to the emotional strains that health care professionals may feel as a result of ambivalence about or disagreement with treatment decisions. Institutional policies should anticipate such developments and provide for mechanisms to address these situations.

Ethics in the Emerging
Health Care Environment

**Health Care Delivery
System Structure**

As this second edition of *Values in Conflict* goes to press, health care delivery is undergoing fundamental change on the community level, and national health care reform is being debated in Congress. Action in Congress could accelerate changes at the community level. However, even in the absence of national health care reform, the momentum for changing health care delivery will continue.

The changes occurring at the community level focus on organization of integrated health care networks, composed of multiple providers—hospitals, physician groups, long-term care providers, and others—serving a defined group of consumers. In the best scenarios, these networks would be clinically and fiscally accountable for delivering high quality care to their enrollees along a seamless continuum and also would be focused on improving the health status of its broader community. Networks would emphasize promotion of health through preventive and primary care services, as opposed to focusing only on illness and acute care services. In some cases, preventive and primary care would be part of the services offered by the hospital; in others, this care would be offered through collaborative arrangements with other providers. The network and the institution would need to periodically review the allocation of resources to determine if their use best meets community and enrollee needs.

While the ethical obligations and imperatives discussed in the previous chapters are the same, the nature of these networks create additional ethical issues and questions for hospitals and their partners in the network. While networks could have many types of arrangements and could vary in their payment structure, many networks, hospitals, and physicians would be paid through a capitated system, which would dramatically change incentives in delivering health care services.

Networks paid on a capitated basis are likely to be responsible for delivering a coordinated continuum of high-quality, appropriate services to their enrollees. Within the constraints of capitation and management of care, networks and hospitals should maintain maximum patient autonomy in choosing services and should ensure that enrollees understand appropriate limitations.

Appropriateness of Care. Because health care resources will be limited in any kind of payment system, networks and hospitals will experience continuing pressure to keep costs down. Although decisions made on the national level may extend a standard benefit package to all persons, decisions as to the appropriateness of care for each individual will continue to be made on a patient-by-patient basis, and decisions about resource allocation among services will be made by individual communities.

Appropriate utilization of resources is particularly important when managing within fixed resources. Emphasis on management of care and resource allocation has moved toward identifying unnecessary or inappropriate care and determining when care will have marginal or no value for particular patients under particular circumstances. To make the most of limited health care resources, hospitals and health care networks should support the development and acceptance of information on patterns of practice, effectiveness, and outcome of care. Lack of information on which treatments make a substantial difference in outcome (both in rarer, high-cost interventions and in routinely applied, lower-cost procedures) makes intelligent resource allocation very difficult. More reliable information on the optimal distribution and use of services such as ICU beds and other high technology services could assist hospitals and networks in tempering unneeded duplication of expensive services and equipment, which raises costs systemwide.

Choice. Capitated networks of care impose limitations on patient choice. It is imperative that consumers understand the limitations as well as the benefits, quality, and other aspects of performance in selecting an integrated network. It is also important that, within the constraints of a managed care environment, the patient's role in decision making be maintained.

The most visible limitation is a person's choice of providers, which may be limited to those within a network, with a primary care physician or other gatekeeper controlling referral to specialists and other health care resources. However, other limitations may be placed through the network's practice protocols or resource allocation decisions.

The increasing use of gatekeepers and the development of practice protocols should emphasize the goal of providing appropriate and coordinated care. However, patients should be made aware of other treatment options that are available and appropriate for their condition. The hospital or network should have policies to ensure that all available options, risks, benefits, and financial implications are shared with the patient to promote fully informed decision making. The hospital or network should also have a well-publicized procedure or mechanism for patient, physicians, and other practitioners to call for reexamination of decisions affecting access to patient care services and stringent quality monitoring procedures to prevent undertreatment of medical conditions.

Other patient choices should be maintained to the extent possible. For example, planning for post-hospital care or at-home support services should involve the patient and family in making choices.

Network Responsibility to Community

Hospitals and health care networks should consider the overall welfare of their communities as well as enrollees in determining the organization's activities and should strive to meet the needs of all segments of the population, including individuals with conditions that are more difficult to treat.

Collaborative Efforts. Health care networks and institutions are responsible for fair and effective use of available health care delivery resources to promote access to comprehensive and affordable health care services of high quality. This responsibility extends beyond the resources of the given network and the care of its enrollees to include efforts to coordinate with other health care organizations and professionals and to share in community solutions for improving overall community health status. If a health care network or a hospital perceives a community need that extends beyond its own enrollees, it should explore joint projects within the community and with other networks.

Full Information. To make informed decisions in selecting networks or providers, people must have access to adequate information on the quality, cost, financial soundness, and enrollee satisfaction of the network or provider. Those choosing a network should be informed about the providers participating in the network, including physicians, hospitals, and other providers.

Information should be available on the financial incentives in network and hospital arrangements. The American Hospital Association's *A Patient's Bill of Rights* supports a patient's right to ask and be informed of the existence of business relationships among the hospital, educational institutions, other health care providers, or payers that may influence the patient's treatment and care. With the proliferation of innovative and unfamiliar payment and delivery systems, providers should continue to ensure that patients can find out about the organizational and financial relationships among their providers.

Health Care Service Decisions

A restructured health care delivery and financing system based on integrated networks and capitated payment holds promise for promoting comprehensiveness of services and continuity of care. It can also present new resource allocation issues.

These questions of resource allocation will have ethical as well as practical and financial components. The answers must take into account the hospital's mission and community needs.

Hospital Mission

While networks must ensure access to all services offered in a health care benefit package, the particular programs, services, and activities of hospitals should embody the health care institution's mission and values as well as community needs. A hospital may choose not to provide a service if the service is incompatible with its mission or clashes with religious values or if other providers adequately meet the need. The hospital has an obligation to inform the community of the institution's mission and services it will not offer.

Special Considerations

New Patient Care Services and Technology. Decisions on starting new patient care services or acquiring new technology should be consistent with the hospital's mission and the availability of the technology within the integrated network, and hospital and network policies should reflect these factors. Typically, even the most promising new technology presents many unknowns regarding costs, safety, efficacy, and efficiency. To the extent that these can be quantified and projected, the hospital should make reasonable efforts to assess them based on available data and, where possible, on the known experience of other institutions. Practices regarding the acquisition of technology should be based on how the acquisition will affect the ability to provide other needed services, whether the technology is adequately available in other facilities, how many individuals will benefit, and how the technology may affect the safety and comfort of patients. Once new technology has been acquired, these factors provide the basis for periodic evaluation and for decisions as to whether to continue providing the service. Before acquiring new technology, the hospital must be certain that its professional staff has the qualifications and competence to properly apply it.

Acquisition of new technology often requires a trade-off between the new and exciting and the more basic. The ethical implications of these trade-offs must be considered. Although major new technology increases the hospital's prestige, this should not be a primary reason for acquiring new equipment. Moreover, because acquisition of high-priced equipment often generates public interest, it may require special attention to privacy and confidentiality for patients.

The way in which cost-effectiveness is considered in technology decisions varies according to the mission of the institution and its role within its network. Teaching and research hospitals involved in testing innovative equipment, drugs, and new procedures, for example, would balance the cost-effectiveness issue differently than would a community hospital. Not all technology is expensive to purchase, but even inexpensive items may result in new procedures and practices with implications of cost, quality of care, exclusion of other services, and human resources, and these should be thoroughly assessed.

Organ Transplantation. Improved surgical techniques, better tissue matching, and the use of new immunosuppressive drugs all have made transplants more feasible. As a result, many institutions are pressured to decide whether transplantation services are appropriate for the hospital and its community.

When making these decisions, the hospital should rely essentially on the same principles as for the acquisition of other new technology. Particular attention should be given to the impact of organ transplantation programs on other hospital services (for example, the increased demand for intensive care unit beds) and the shifting of resources away from meeting other, more common health care needs of the community. Hospitals and networks should also consider whether the need for an organ transplant program is already being met by other hospitals that are part of or can contract with the network.

The effort to allocate organs fairly is monitored by a national nonprofit organization under contract with the federal government. United Network for Organ Sharing (UNOS) promulgates regulations regarding criteria for procurement, listing, and transplantation. To ensure equitable access to scarce organs by all patients and regions, hospitals should comply with listing guidelines and national policies regarding procurement and transplantation. This is a domain in which independently developed hospital policies may threaten fair allocation of resources.

Intensive Care Units. Sometimes resources must be allocated within the hospital service or unit. For example, a pool of intensive care beds must be distributed among those needing special care. These decisions are often made by an individual or committee attempting to balance competing needs of many patients. The Joint Commission on Accreditation of Healthcare Organizations *Accreditation Manual for Hospitals, 1994* requires that special care units have written criteria for patient admission and discharge, including priority determination, and that the written criteria are developed by the medical staff with the participation of the nursing department or service.

Hospitals and networks should ensure that these scarce resources are distributed in an ethical way—that the written criteria are just and fairly applied. Consultation with the hospital's ethics committee should be available both in drafting criteria and in helping caregivers and individual patients in making decisions when questions and differences of interpretation arise.

Health Care's Future Environment

The challenge of dealing with biomedical ethics within health care and within society continually grows more complex. This report has attempted to provide guidance to help hospitals and networks develop policies and procedures to resolve the ethical questions that arise in delivery of patient care. Although tomorrow's challenges might be completely new, they will likely be extensions of today's challenges. Developing scientific, technological, and societal forces will bring health care providers face-to-face with amplified biomedical ethics issues. To be prepared, hospitals and networks should develop some type of mechanism to help them identify biomedical ethical issues not yet foreseen in today's environment, to foster discussion about them, and to develop policies and procedures for addressing those issues as they emerge.

Although policies and procedures on various issues in biomedical ethics will differ, they must stress two elements: awareness and communication. Heightening the awareness of everyone in health care delivery of ethical dimensions of patient care and encouraging open communication concerning policies, incidents, and problems relating to ethics are essential to an effective institution-wide and networkwide approach to biomedical ethics.

Genetics

The scientific progress of the Human Genome Project, research to map human genetics, will be translated into the care of patients. Once gene markers are identified, testing can reveal an individual's potential for developing a disease or for passing on a disease to offspring. Perhaps, new forms of gene therapy or gene manipulation will alleviate symptoms or progression of diseases caused by damaged or defective genes.

Society as well as health care providers will need to wrestle with issues raised by progress in human genetics, including the impact of genetic counseling on individuals and on reproductive decisions. Society will also be called on to deal with the use of genetic knowledge to select characteristics or enhance traits unrelated to defective genes.

Health care providers will need to determine what genetic tests to offer, set priorities among tests, counsel persons who are undergoing genetic screening, and protect results from unauthorized disclosure. As genetic screening and treatment progress, hospitals and networks will need to develop policies and procedures and support the education of geneticists and other physicians and health care professionals who will encounter and work with these advances in human genetics.

Confidentiality	Continued technological developments in information processing and transfer will vastly increase the amount and accessibility of information about patients and their care. Hospitals and networks must take special care in safeguarding information while still making useful information available to patients, payers, and others, where appropriate.
Assisted Suicide	Long-standing legal and professional prohibitions against medical personnel assisting a patient in suicide may soon come into conflict with state measures allowing assisted suicide for terminally ill patients within prescribed criteria. If assisted suicide is legalized within a state, hospitals, physicians, and networks must be prepared to develop policies and procedures complying with state law and respectful of professional codes of ethics. Because interest in legalizing assisted suicide often stems from individuals' concerns about prolonged pain, abandonment, and loss of dignity, hospitals and networks should strive to continually improve pain management, palliative care, and hospice services.
Cultural Diversity	Health care professionals and hospital staffs will find new challenges in communicating with patients and respecting their varied cultural and healing beliefs. Patients and their families will likely demand coexistence of mainstream medicine with traditional healing processes from various cultures or with nontraditional alternative medicine. Likewise, cultural diversity will increase in the health care workplace, and health care employers will strive to meet and respect employees' needs. Growing multiculturalism in the patient population and the health care work force might heighten the impact of cultural, ethnic, and religious differences.
Provider-Patient Relationships	Current questions surrounding the roles and relationships of providers and patients will likely intensify in the future. Questions raised in today's debate on futility of care as to when patient or surrogate choices are not appropriate likely will be magnified in the future. Continuation of medical advances likely will perpetuate unrealistic and inappropriate expectations of medical care—perhaps fostered by health care providers, media reports of miracle cures, or societal wishes for a quick and painless technological fix for poor health habits. Equally likely, as the

health care delivery and financing system change, the roles and responsibilities of providers will change. These conflicts, disappointed expectations, and role changes might impact providers' relationships with patients and their families or with other providers.

The Environment and Health Care

The domain of health care is already much larger than medical care. Providers are realizing that sometimes the greatest determinant of a person's health status may be nutrition or education, a job, or housing. Other even broader factors also demonstrably influence the health of a person or a community, including pollutants in the water, air, and soil. In the future, hospitals and health networks may find themselves involved in the intersection of biomedical ethics with environmental ethics—in pushing the frontiers of prevention into local and global pollution or other ecosystem matters.

Conclusion

Hospitals and health care networks cannot be passive in the face of such future challenges. They must work individually, together, and through their associations to resolve institutional and community-level issues. They must take the lead in drawing national attention to ethical concerns that should be discussed and debated openly in the broadest public policy arenas.

Dealing with the differing values inherent in biomedical ethics is an ongoing process for health care networks, hospitals, and health care professionals. As medical knowledge continues to expand, social priorities and emphasis continue to shift, and individuals continue to raise fundamental concerns about the ethics of health care treatment and delivery, health care networks and hospitals will need policies and procedures to guide resolution of biomedical ethical questions.

It is the moral responsibility of each health care network and hospital to recognize and respond to such questions. Certainly, much remains to be done. This report is an attempt to provide a framework to increase awareness and to stimulate discussion of biomedical ethics in the hospital and the health care network.

Appendix A

Roster of the American Hospital Association
Technical Panel on Biomedical Ethics

Chairman

Paul B. Hofmann is visiting scholar, Stanford University Center for Biomedical Ethics, Palo Alto. Hofmann previously served as executive vice president and chief operating officer of the Alta Bates Corporation, a diversified health care system in Northern California. In the past, he held appointments as executive director of Emory University Hospital and director of Stanford University Hospital and Clinics. He is a fellow of the American College of Healthcare Executives and serves as its consultant in health care management ethics. He is on the board of the International Bioethics Institute and a member of the Ethics Task Force of the Society of Critical Care Medicine. He is also a doctoral candidate in health policy and administration at the University of California, Berkeley, from which he received his bachelor and master of public health degrees.

Members

Jean Adnopoz is an associate clinical professor in the Yale Child Study Center, Yale University School of Medicine, and the clinical coordinator of the Center's Community Child Development Programs. She is chairperson of the Advisory Council to the Connecticut Department of Children and Families and a member of the National Crime Prevention Council. She is a past vice-chairman of the Board of Directors of Yale-New Haven Hospital and past chairman of the Connecticut Hospital Association. She received her bachelor's degree from Wellesley College, Wellesley, Massachusetts, and a master's degree from the Department of Epidemiology and Public Health, Yale University School of Medicine.

Nancy Green is director of the Patient Relations Department of the University of Minnesota Health System. Serving as a patient advocate for 18 years, she now directs a department that supports and educates patients, families, and staff in patient rights, advance directives, and ethics. She co-chairs the health system's bioethics committee and coordinates ethics consults. A fellow of the National Society of Patient Representation and Consumer Affairs, she is the organization's past president. She received her degree from the University of Minnesota.

Robert L. Harman is administrator of Grant Memorial Hospital in Petersburg, West Virginia. His participation in the American Hospital Association includes chairing the Section for Small or Rural Hospitals. He has served as chairman of the West Virginia Hospital Association. He received his bachelor's degree in business administration from Fairmont State College in Fairmont, West Virginia, and master's degree in health care administration from George Washington University.

Bruce Jennings is executive director of The Hastings Center, where he has directed several research projects on professional ethics, health policy, chronic illness, long-term care, and the care of the terminally ill. He has written and edited nine book, published numerous articles on bioethics and public policy issues, and served as a consultant to several governmental and private organizations. A political scientist by training, Jennings received a bachelor's degree from Yale University and a master's degree from Princeton University.

Joanne Lynn, M.D., is professor of medicine and of community and family medicine, associate director of the Center for the Aging, and senior associate in the Center for the Evaluative Clinical Sciences, Dartmouth Medical School, Dartmouth-Hitchcock Medical Center. She chairs the Ethics Committee and serves on the board of directors and Committee on Public Policy of the American Geriatrics Society, is a member of the Institute of Medicine Committee on the Social and Ethical Impacts of Advances in Biomedicine, and serves on the Geriatrics and Gerontology Advisory Committee to the Department of Veterans Affairs and on the Veterans Health Administration National Bioethics Committee. Dr. Lynn received her medical degree from Boston University and her master's degree in philosophy and social policy from George Washington University.

Ruth Macklin, Ph.D., heads the Division of Philosophy and History of Medicine, Department of Epidemiology and Social Medicine, at Albert Einstein College of Medicine, Bronx, New York. She is also a professor of bioethics and the Shoshanah Trachtenberg Frackman Faculty Scholar in biomedical ethics. She is on the board of directors of the American Association of Bioethics, vice chairman of the National Advisory Board on Ethics in Reproduction, and author of several books, most recently *Surrogates and Other Mothers: The Debates over Assisted Reproduction* and *Enemies of Patients*. She graduated from Cornell University with distinction and received a master's and doctorate in philosophy from Case Western Reserve University.

Christine Mitchell, R.N., is a fellow in the Program in Ethics and the Professions at Harvard University during 1993 and 1994, on leave from Children's Hospital, Boston, where she is the hospital ethicist, co-chairs the Ethics Advisory Committee, and advises the Nursing Ethics Committee. She is also an ethics consultant to the departments of nursing at Massachusetts General Hospital and New England Deaconess Hospital. A fellow of the American Academy of Nursing, she served on the American Nurses Association Committee on Ethics and is a director of the Society for Bioethics Consultation and former president of the American Society of Law, Medicine and Ethics. She is a doctoral candidate at Boston College, having received a master's in Ethics from Harvard University and master's and bachelor's degrees in nursing from Boston University.

Robyn S. Shapiro, J.D., is director of the Center for the Study of Bioethics, Medical College of Wisconsin, Milwaukee, and a partner in the Health Care Practice Group of Michael, Best & Friedrich. She also served on the American Hospital Association Ad Hoc Committee on AIDS Policy, as well as local, state, and national organizations on biomedical ethics, including the national advisory committee of Health Decisions USA. Currently, she directs the Ethics Committee Task Force of the International Association of Bioethics. She graduated summa cum laude from the University of Michigan, Ann Arbor, and received her law degree from Harvard Law School, Cambridge, Massachusetts.

Kenneth A. Shull is president of Lexington Medical Center, West Columbia, South Carolina. He has served as chairman of the American Hospital Association Section for Small or Rural Hospitals and as chairman of the South Carolina Hospital Association Board of Trustees. Shull is a fellow of the American College of Healthcare Executives. He received a bachelor's degree in biology from Denison University, Granville, Ohio; a master's degree in business administration from Southern Illinois University at Edwardsville; and a master's degree in hospital administration from the Medical College of Virginia/Virginia Commonwealth University, Richmond.

Staff

Gail M. Lovinger, secretary to the Technical Panel on Biomedical Ethics, is director, Association Governance and assistant secretary of the American Hospital Association. Ms. Lovinger staffed AHA's Special Committee on Biomedical Ethics in 1984-1985 and was a principal writer of the first edition of Values in Conflict. She received her master's degree in speech communication from the University of Illinois, Champaign-Urbana and attended the Intensive Bioethics Course at the Kennedy Institute of Ethics, Georgetown University.

Kathy E. Poole, assistant secretary to the Technical Panel on Biomedical Ethics, is senior staff specialist, Office of the Secretary, American Hospital Association. She has written and edited books, magazines, newsletters, speeches, and other communications on health care, business, and public policy. She received a bachelors degree from the University of Kansas and studied linguistics at the University of Chicago.

Appendix B

A Patient's Bill of Rights

Introduction

Effective health care requires collaboration between patients and physicians and other health care professionals. Open and honest communication, respect for personal and professional values, and sensitivity to differences are integral to optimal patient care. As the setting for the provision of health services, hospitals must provide a foundation for understanding and respecting the rights and responsibilities of patients, their families, physicians, and other caregivers. Hospitals must ensure a health care ethic that respects the role of patients in decision making about treatment choices and other aspects of their care. Hospitals must be sensitive to cultural, racial, linguistic, religious, age, gender, and other differences as well as the needs of persons with disabilities.

The American Hospital Association presents *A Patient's Bill of Rights* with the expectation that it will contribute to more effective patient care and be supported by the hospital on behalf of the institution, its medical staff, employees, and patients. The American Hospital Association encourages health care institutions to tailor this bill of rights to their patient community by translating and/or simplifying the language of this bill of rights as may be necessary to ensure that patients and their families understand their rights and responsibilities.

Bill of Rights*

*These rights can be exercised on the patient's behalf by a designated surrogate or proxy decision maker if the patient lacks decision-making capacity, is legally incompetent, or is a minor.

1. The patient has the right to considerate and respectful care.
2. The patient has the right to and is encouraged to obtain from physicians and other direct caregivers relevant, current, and understandable information concerning diagnosis, treatment, and prognosis.

   Except in emergencies when the patient lacks decision-making capacity and the need for treatment is urgent, the patient is entitled to the opportunity to discuss and request information related to the specific procedures and/or treatments, the risks involved, the possible length of recuperation, and the medically reasonable alternatives and their accompanying risks and benefits.

Patients have the right to know the identity of physicians, nurses, and others involved in their care, as well as when those involved are students, residents, or other trainees. The patient also has the right to know the immediate and long-term financial implications of treatment choices, insofar as they are known.

3. The patient has the right to make decisions about the plan of care prior to and during the course of treatment and to refuse a recommended treatment or plan of care to the extent permitted by law and hospital policy and to be informed of the medical consequences of this action. In case of such refusal, the patient is entitled to other appropriate care and services that the hospital provides or transfer to another hospital. The hospital should notify patients of any policy that might affect patient choice within the institution.

4. The patient has the right to have an advance directive (such as a living will, health care proxy, or durable power of attorney for health care) concerning treatment or designating a surrogate decision maker with the expectation that the hospital will honor the intent of that directive to the extent permitted by law and hospital policy.

   Health care institutions must advise patients of their rights under state law and hospital policy to make informed medical choices, ask if the patient has an advance directive, and include that information in patient records. The patient has the right to timely information about hospital policy that may limit its ability to implement fully a legally valid advance directive.

5. The patient has the right to every consideration of privacy. Case discussion, consultation, examination, and treatment should be conducted so as to protect each patient's privacy.

6. The patient has the right to expect that all communications and records pertaining to his/her care will be treated as confidential by the hospital, except in cases such as suspected abuse and public health hazards when reporting is permitted or required by law. The patient has the right to expect that the hospital will emphasize the confidentiality of this information when it releases it to any other parties entitled to review information in these records.

7. The patient has the right to review the records pertaining to his/her medical care and to have the information explained or interpreted as necessary, except when restricted by law.

8. The patient has the right to expect that, within its capacity and policies, a hospital will make reasonable response to the request of a patient for appropriate and medically indicated care and services. The hospital must provide evaluation, service, and/or referral as indicated by the urgency of the case. When medically appropriate and legally permissible, or when a patient has so requested, a patient may be transferred to another facility. The institution to which the patient is to be transferred must first have accepted the patient for transfer. The patient must also have the benefit of complete information and explanation concerning the need for, risks, benefits, and alternatives to such a transfer.

9. The patient has the right to ask and be informed of the existence of business relationships among the hospital, educational institutions, other health care providers, or payers that may influence the patient's treatment and care.

10. The patient has the right to consent to or decline to participate in proposed research studies or human experimentation affecting care and treatment or requiring direct patient involvement, and to have those studies fully explained prior to consent. A patient who declines to participate in research or experimentation is entitled to the most effective care that the hospital can otherwise provide.

11. The patient has the right to expect reasonable continuity of care when appropriate and to be informed by physicians and other caregivers of available and realistic patient care options when hospital care is no longer appropriate.

12. The patient has the right to be informed of hospital policies and practices that relate to patient care, treatment, and responsibilities. The patient has the right to be informed of available resources for resolving disputes, grievances, and conflicts, such as ethics committees, patient representatives, or other mechanisms available in the institution. The patient has the right to be informed of the hospital's charges for services and available payment methods.

The collaborative nature of health care requires that patients, or their families/surrogates, participate in their care. The effectiveness of care and patient satisfaction with the course of treatment depend, in part, on the patient fulfilling certain responsibilities. Patients are responsible for providing information about past illnesses, hospitalizations, medications, and other matters related to health status. To participate effectively in decision making, patients must be encouraged to take responsibility for requesting additional information or clarification about their health status or treatment when they do not fully understand information and instructions. Patients are also responsible for ensuring that the health care institution has a copy of their written advance directive if they have one. Patients are responsible for informing their physicians and other caregivers if they anticipate problems in following prescribed treatment.

Patients should also be aware of the hospital's obligation to be reasonably efficient and equitable in providing care to other patients and the community. The hospital's rules and regulations are designed to help the hospital meet this obligation. Patients and their families are responsible for making reasonable accommodations to the needs of the hospital, other patients, medical staff, and hospital employees. Patients are responsible for providing necessary information for insurance claims and for working with the hospital to make payment arrangements, when necessary.

A person's health depends on much more than health care services. Patients are responsible for recognizing the impact of their life-style on their personal health.

Conclusion

Hospitals have many functions to perform, including the enhancement of health status, health promotion, and the prevention and treatment of injury and disease; the immediate and ongoing care and rehabilitation of patients; the education of health professionals, patients, and the community; and research. All these activities must be conducted with an overriding concern for the values and dignity of patients.

Selected Recommended Resources and Readings

General

American College of Physicians ethics manual. 3rd ed. *Annals of Internal Medicine*. 117: 947-960, 1992.

Annas, G. J. *The Rights of Patients*. 2nd ed. Carbondale and Edwardsville: Southern Illinois University Press, 1989.

Beauchamp, T. L., and Childress, J. F. *Principles of Biomedical Ethics*. 3rd ed. New York City: Oxford University Press, 1989.

Benjamin, M., and Curtis, J. *Ethics in Nursing*. 3rd ed. New York City: Oxford University Press, 1992.

BIOETHICS (Online Data Base). Available through MEDLARS computer systems of National Library of Medicine. Produced by Kennedy Institute of Ethics, Georgetown University, Washington, DC.

Friedman, E. ed. *Making Choices: Ethics Issues for Health Care Professionals*. Chicago: American Hospital Publishing, 1986.

Friedman, E. ed. *Choices and Conflict: Explorations in Health Care Ethics*. Chicago: American Hospital Publishing, 1992.

Garrett, T. M., Baillie, H. W., and Garrett, R. M. *Health Care Ethics: Principles and Problems*. Englewood Cliffs, NJ: Prentice Hall, 1989.

Griffith, J. R. *The Moral Challenges of Health Care Management*. Ann Arbor, MI: Health Administration Press, 1993.

Ingelfinger, F. I. Arrogance. *New England Journal of Medicine*. 303(26):1507-1511, December 25, 1980.

Jonsen, Albert R. et al. *Clinical Ethics: A Practical Approach to Ethical Decisions in Clinical Medicine.* 3rd ed. New York City: MacGraw, 1992.

Levine, C. *Taking Sides*, 4th ed. Guilford, CT: Dushkin Publishing Group, Inc., 1991.

Macklin, R. *Mortal Choices: Ethical Dilemmas in Modern Medicine.* Boston: Houghton Mifflin Company, 1988.

National Center for State Courts. *Guidelines for State Court Decision Making in Authorizing or Withholding Life-Sustaining Medical Treatment.* St. Paul: West Publishing Company, 1991.

President's Commission for the Study of Ethical Problems in Medicine and Biomedical and Behavioral Research. *Deciding to Forego Life-Sustaining Treatment* (1983); *Defining Death* (1981); and *Making Health Care Decisions* (1982). Washington, DC: U.S. Government Printing Office.

Reich, W. T. ed. *Encyclopedia of Bioethics.* New York City: The Free Press, 1978. Second Edition in press.

Society of Critical Care Medicine. Consensus Statement on the Triage of Critically Ill Patients. Anaheim, CA: SCCM, 1993.

Zucker, A., Borchert, D., and Stewart, D. ed. *Medical Ethics: A Reader.* Englewood Cliffs, NJ: Prentice Hall, 1992.

Case Studies

Cohen, C. B. ed. *Casebook on the Termination of Life-Sustaining Treatment and Care of the Dying*, Bloomington, IN: Indiana University Press, 1988.

Crigger, B. ed. *Cases in Bioethics: Selections from the Hastings Center Report.* 2nd ed. New York City: St. Martin's Press, 1993.

Periodicals

Bioethics. Cambridge, MA: Blackwell Publishers.

Cambridge Quarterly of Healthcare Ethics. New York City: Cambridge University Press.

Ethical Currents. Center for Healthcare Ethics, Orange, CA: St. Joseph Health Systems.

Hastings Center Report. Briarcliff Manor, NY: The Hastings Center.

Hospital Ethics. Chicago: American Hospital Association.

The Journal of Clinical Ethics. Frederick, MD: University Publishing Group.

The Journal of Law, Medicine & Ethics. Boston: American Society of Law, Medicine & Ethics.

Kennedy Institute of Ethics Journal. Baltimore: John Hopkins University Press.

Care of the Dying

Doyle, D., Hanks, G. W. C., and MacDonald, N. ed. *Oxford Textbook of Palliative Medicine.* New York: Oxford University Press, 1993.

The Hastings Center. *Guidelines on the Termination of Life-Sustaining Treatment and the Care of the Dying.* Bloomington: Indiana University Press, 1988.

Hofmann, P. Decisions near the end of life: resource allocation implications for hospitals. *Cambridge Quarterly of Healthcare Ethics.* 1(3):229-237, Summer 1992.

Lynn, J., and Childress, J. Must patients always be given food and water. *The Hastings Center Report.* 13(5):17-21, October 1983.

Johnson, D. Helga Wanglie revisited: medical futility and the limits of autonomy. *Cambridge Quarterly of Healthcare Ethics.* 2(2):161-170, Spring 1993.

Massachusetts General Hospital Clinical Care Committee. Optimum care for hopelessly ill patients. *New England Journal of Medicine.* 295(7):362-364, August 12, 1976.

President's Commission for the Study of Ethical Problems in Medicine and Biomedical and Behavioral Research. *Deciding to Forego Life-Sustaining Treatment.* Washington, DC: U.S. Government Printing Office, 1983.

President's Commission for the Study of Ethical Problems in Medicine and Biomedical and Behavioral Research. *Defining Death.* Washington, DC: U.S. Government Printing Office, 1981.

Sabatino, F. Easing passages: a hospital's policy on life-sustaining treatment. *Trustee,* 44(10):4-5, 21, 44, October 1991.

Confidentiality

Alpert, S. Smart cards, smarter policy: medical records, privacy, and health care reform. *Hastings Center Report* 23(6):13-23, November-December 1993.

Bruce, J. C. *Privacy and Confidentiality of Health Care Information.* 2nd ed. Chicago: American Hospital Publishing. 1988.

Decision Making

Buchanan, A. E., and Brock, D. W. *Deciding for Others.* New York City: Cambridge University Press, 1987.

DeGrazia, D., and Lynn, J. An outcomes model of medical decision-making. *Journal of Theoretical Medicine* (now *Journal of Medicine and Philosophy*). 12:325-342, 1991.

Jackson, D. L., and Youngner, S. Patient autonomy and "death with dignity": some clinical caveats. *New England Journal of Medicine.* 301(8):404-8, August 23, 1979.

Paridy, N. Complying with the Patient Self-Determination Act: legal, ethical and practical challenges for hospitals. *Hospital & Health Services Administration.* 38(2):287-296, Summer 1993.

President's Commission for the Study of Ethical Problems in Medicine and Biomedical and Behavioral Research. *Making Health Care Decisions: The Ethical and Legal Implications of Informed Consent in the Patient-Practitioner Relationship.* Washington, DC: U.S. Government Printing Office, 1982.

Robertson, J. A. *The Rights of the Critically Ill* (revised ACLU Guide to the Rights of the Critically Ill and Dying Patients). New York City: Bantam Books, 1983.

Disclosure

Bok, S. Impaired physicians: what should patients know? *Cambridge Quarterly of Healthcare Ethics*. 1993(2):331-340, 1993.

Ethics Committees

Agich, G. J., and Youngner, S. J. For experts only? Access to hospital ethics committees. *Hastings Center Report*. 21(4):18-21, 1991.

Purtilo, R. B. Sounding board: ethics consultation in the hospital. *New England Journal of Medicine*. 311(5):983-86, 1984.

Ross, J., Glaser, J., Rasinski-Gregory, D., Gibson, J., and Bayley, C. *Health Care Ethics Committees: The Next Generation*. Chicago: American Hospital Publishing, 1993.

Tulsky, J. A., and Lo, B. Editorial: Ethics consultation: time to focus on patients. *American Journal of Medicine*. 92(4):343-45, 1992.

Wolf, S. M. Toward a theory of process. *Law, Medicine & Health Care*. 20(4):278-90, 1992.

Wolf, S.M. Ethics committees and due process: nesting rights in a community of caring. *Maryland Law Review*. 50(3):798-858, 1991.

Futility

Drane, J. F., and Coulehan, J. L. The concept of futility: patients do not have the right to demand medically useless treatment. *Health Progress*. 74(10):21, 28-32, December 1993.

Veatch, R. M., and Spicer, C. M. Futile care: physicians should not be allowed to refuse to treat. *Health Progress*. 74(10):21-27, December 1993.

Informed Consent

Faden, R. R. and Beauchamp, T. L. *A History and Theory of Informed Consent*. New York City: Oxford University Press, 1986.

Moral Convictions

MacIntyre, A. *Whose Justice? Which Rationality?* Notre Dame, IN: University of Notre Dame Press, 1989.

Walker, M. Keeping moral space open: new images of ethics consulting. *The Hastings Center Report.* 23(2):33-40, March-April 1993.

Rationing

Aaron, H. J., and Schwartz, W. B. *The Painful Prescription: Rationing Hospital Care.* Washington, DC: The Brookings Institution, 1984.

Avorn, J. Benefit and cost analysis in geriatric care. *New England Journal of Medicine.* 310:1294-1301, 1984.

Callahan, D. *Setting Limits.* New York City: Simon & Schuster, 1987.

Callahan, D. *What Kind of Life?* New York City: Simon & Schuster, 1990.

Catholic Health Association. *With Justice for All? The Ethics of Healthcare Rationing.* St. Louis: CHA, 1991.

Daniels, N. *Just Health Care.* New York City: Cambridge University Press, 1985.

Dougherty, C. Ethical problems in healthcare rationing. *Health Progress.* 72(8):32-39, October 1991.

Truog, R. D. Triage in the ICU. *Hastings Center Report.* 22(3):13-17, 1992.

Technology/Transplants

Fox, R. C., and Swazey, J. P. *Spare Parts.* Chicago: University of Chicago Press, 1992.

Fox, R. C., and Swazey, J. P. *The Courage to Fail: A Social View of Organ Transplants and Dialysis.* Chicago: University of Chicago Press, 1978.

Institute of Medicine. *Medical Innovation at the Crossroads.* Vol. 1. *Modern Methods of Clinical Investigation.* Vol. 2. *The Changing Economics of Medical Technology.* Vol. 3. *Technology and Health Care in an Era of Limits.* Washington, DC: IOM, 1992.

Office of Technology Assessment. *Life-Sustaining Technologies and the Elderly.* Washington, DC: U.S. Government Printing Office, 1987.